I0838819

The Ultimate Mediterranean Diet Cookbook 2023

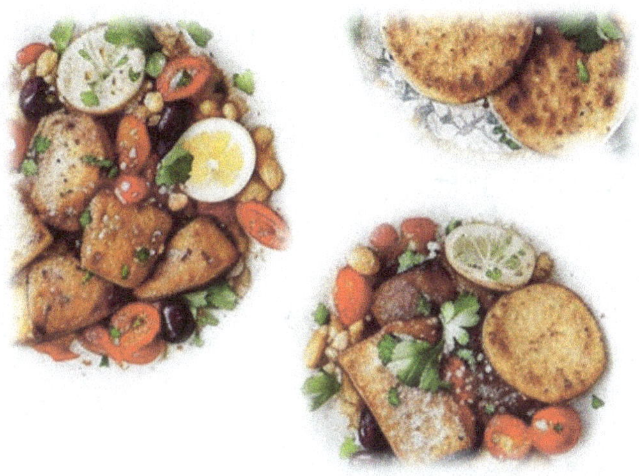

Quick and Easy Healthy Recipes for Beginners

Blessing Dorothy

Copyright © 2023 by Blessing Dorothy

All rights reserved. No part of this book may be reproduced, stored in a retrieval system, or transmitted, in any form or by any means, without the prior written permission of the publisher, except in the case of brief quotations embodied in critical reviews and certain other noncommercial uses permitted by copyright law.

Every effort has been made to ensure that the information in this book is accurate and up-to-date. However, the author and publisher make no warranties or representations, express or implied, as to the accuracy or completeness of the contents of this book.

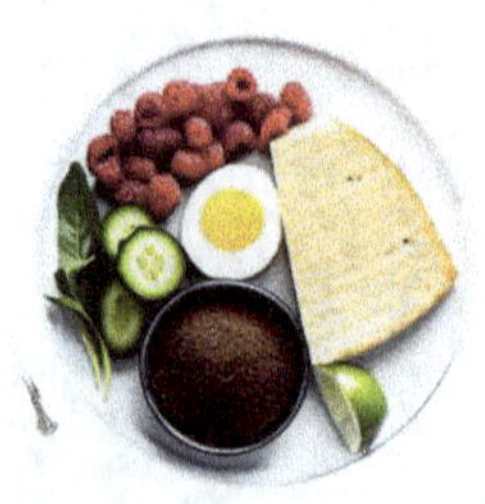

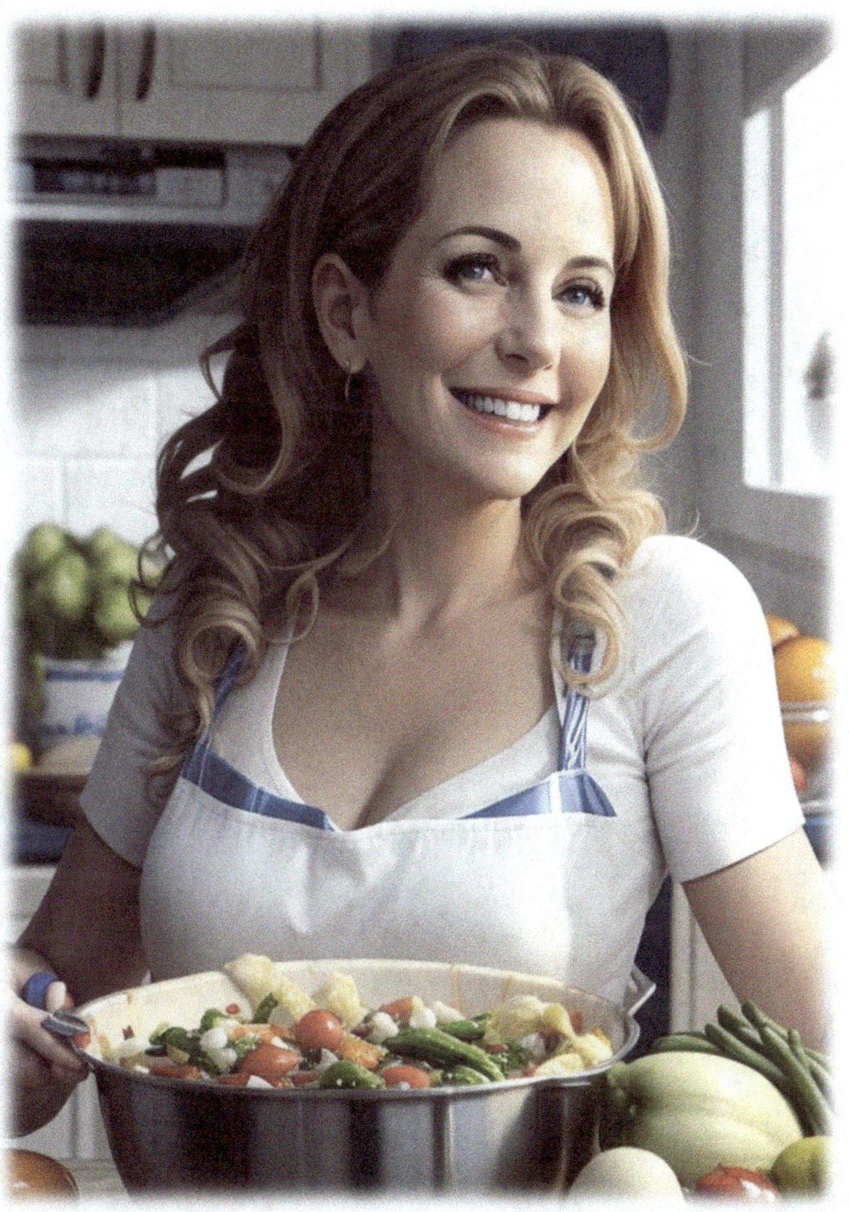

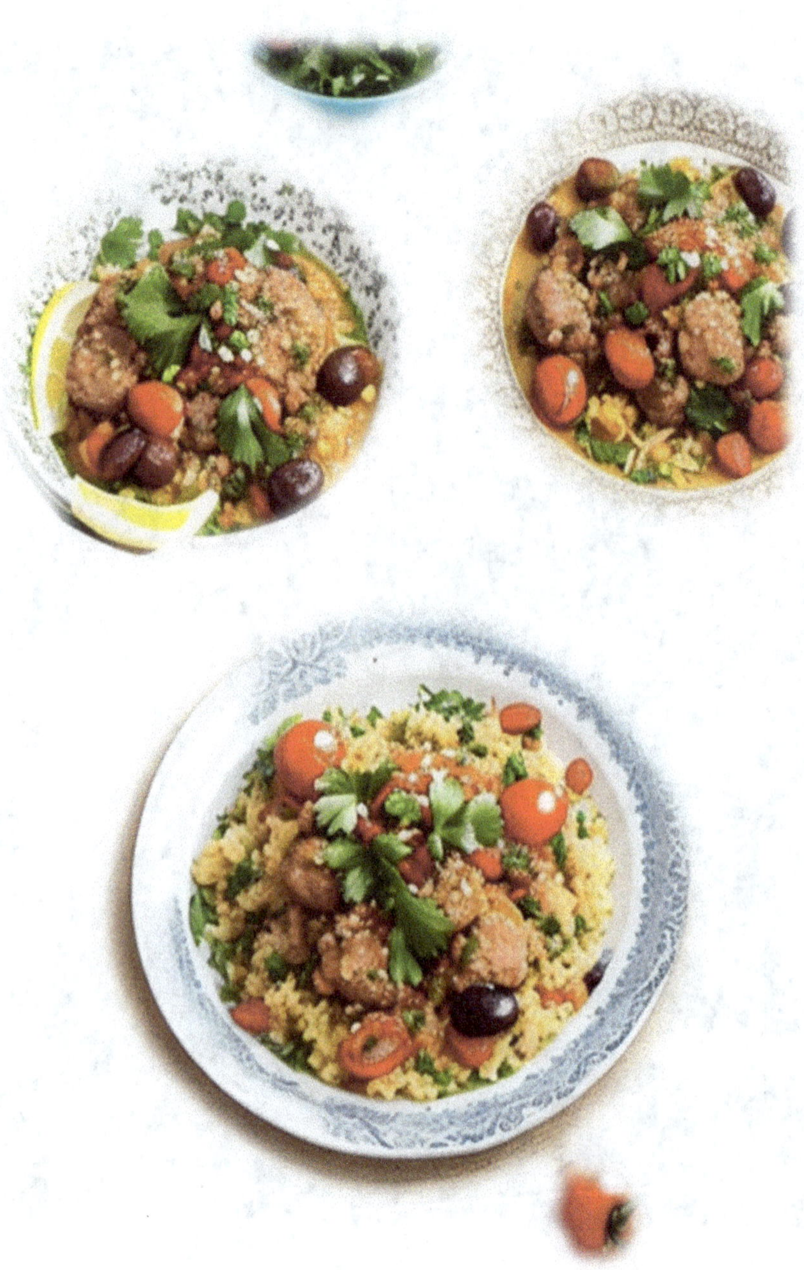

TABLE OF CONTENTS

Introduction

The Mediterranean diet is not just another fad—it's a time-tested, delectable style of eating that provides awesome health benefits. This technique of cooking has been mastered over generations in the sunny Mediterranean area.

Trust me, once you have a taste of these scrumptious fresh foods, you'll feel like you're resting on vacation even while you're cooking at home!

The Mediterranean foods we're discussing here include delicious seafood, vivid vegetable meals, savory herbs, brilliant red wines, and yes, even delectable cheeses.

They provide a robust dose of antioxidants, healthy fats, and lean proteins which our body systems desire.

All that deliciousness not only generates awe-inspiring tastes, but research indicates it may do wonders for your heart, and your waistline, decreasing your chance of chronic diseases down the road. Now that's what I call a win-win!

Transitioning your cuisine to include more of these Mediterranean staples is simpler than you think! Start by filling your kitchen with things like olive oil, almonds, nutritious grains, and fresh veggies.

Then try my simple, delectable recipes for bringing the tastes of the Mediterranean home to your dinner table. With a touch of imagination and a dash of enthusiasm, you'll be mastering this enjoyable, health-boosting style of eating in no time. Get ready to impress your taste buds and your doctor!

Breakfast Recipes

1. Breakfast Tacos

Ingredients:

4 eggs (280 calories)
1/2 onion, diced (15 calories)
1/2 bell pepper, diced (20 calories)
1/2 15-oz can of black beans, rinsed and drained (200 calories)
4 corn tortillas (120 calories)
2 Tbsp salsa (10 calories)
1/4 avocado, sliced (60 calories)
Cilantro

Instructions:

- Add bell pepper and onion to scrambled eggs.
- Warm up the tortillas.
- To assemble tacos, layer tortillas with salsa, black beans, scrambled eggs, avocado slices, and cilantro.

Total Calories: 705 calories

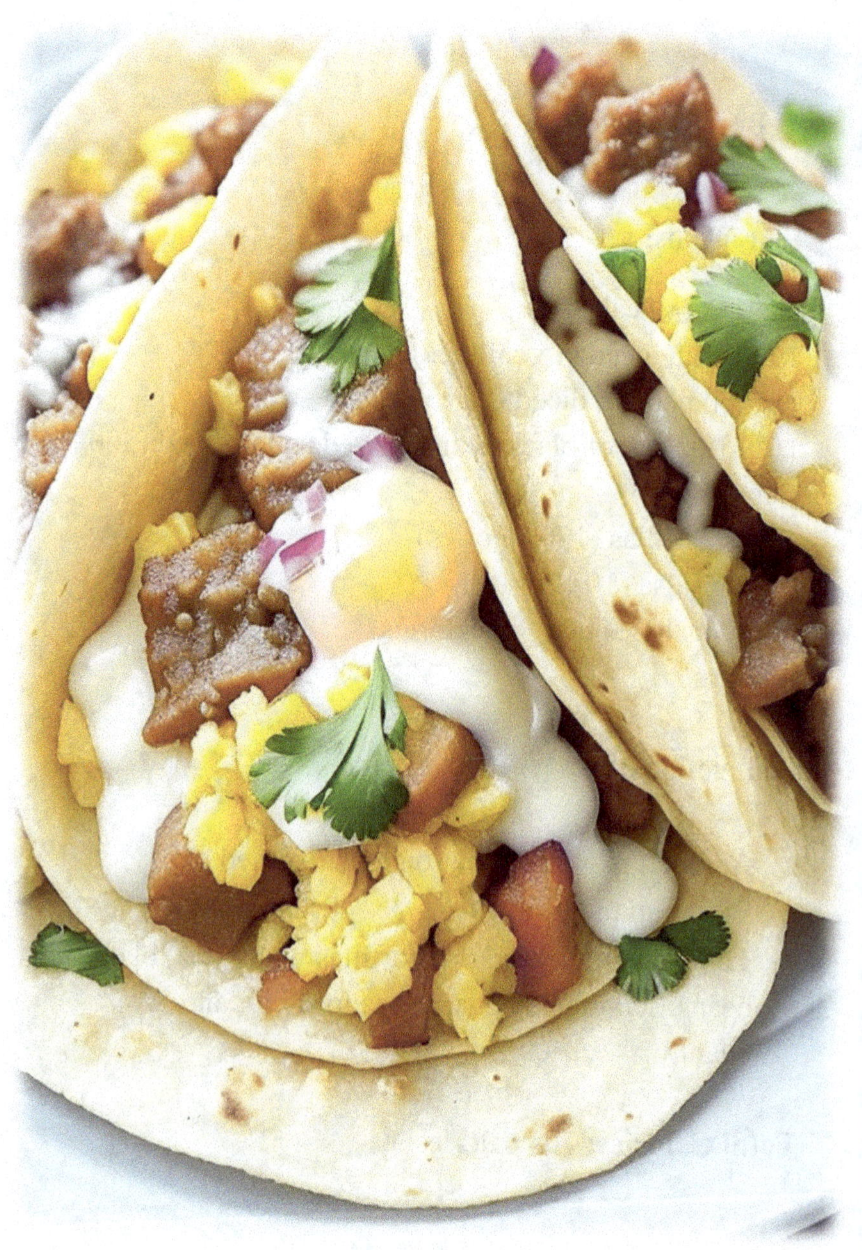

2. Vegetable Frittata

Ingredients:

6 eggs (420 calories)
1 cup baby spinach (20 calories)
1/2 cup cherry tomatoes (30 calories)
2 Tbsp crumbled feta cheese (40 calories)
1 tsp olive oil (40 calories)
Salt and pepper to taste

Instructions:

- Warm the oven to about 375 degrees.
- In a skillet that can be used in the oven, heat the olive oil.
- Cook the spinach and tomatoes for an additional two to three minutes, or until the spinach is wilted.
- Eggs should be beaten with salt and pepper in a bowl.
- Over the vegetable assortment in the skillet, pour the eggs.
- Feta cheese should be added on top.
- Swelter for 12 to 15 minutes, or till the frittata is set.
- Slice and serve after allowing to slightly cool.

Total Calories: 550

3. Overnight Oats

Ingredients:

1/2 cup rolled oats (150 calories)
1/2 cup milk of choice (80 calories for 2% milk)
1 Tbsp chia seeds (70 calories)
1 tsp cinnamon
1/2 cup mixed berries (40 calories)

Instructions:

- Combine the milk, oats, chia seeds, and cinnamon in a container. Mix thoroughly.
- Allow it to stay through the night in the refrigerator; covered.
- Place a layer of mixed berries on top in the morning and eat.

Total Calories: 340

4. Avocado Toast

Ingredients:

1 slice of toasted whole-grain bread (100 calories)
1/2 avocado, mashed (120 calories)
1 fried egg (70 calories)
Red pepper flakes
Lemon juice

Instructions:

- Lemon juice, avocado, salt, and pepper should all be combined in a small bowl.
- Use a spoon to gently mash.
- Place the avocado mixture and fried egg on top of the bread toast.
- Add desired toppings or drizzle with olive oil.

Total Calories: 290

5. Greek Yogurt Bowl

Ingredients:

1 cup plain Greek yogurt (150 calories)
1/2 cup mixed berries (40 calories)
1 Tbsp chopped walnuts (45 calories)
1 tsp honey (20 calories)

Instruction:

- Add mixed berries, walnuts, and honey to the Greek yogurt as garnishes.

Total Calories: 255

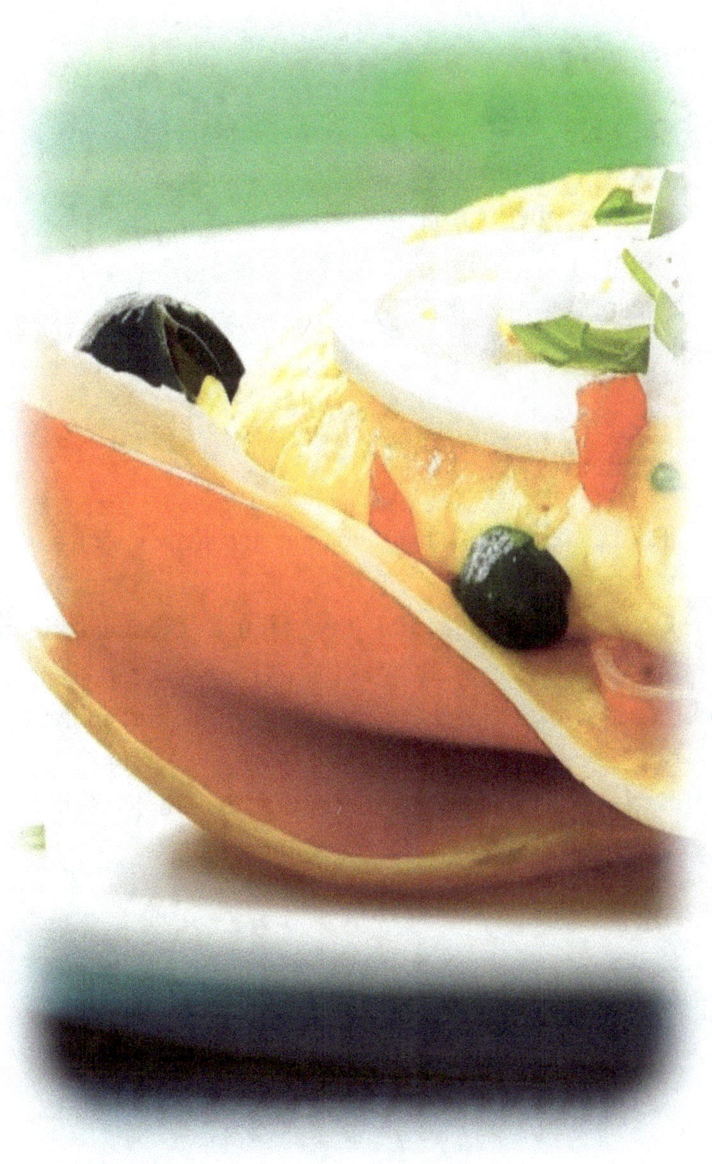

6. Mediterranean Omelets

Ingredients:

3 large eggs
1/4 cup diced tomatoes
1/4 cup chopped spinach
1/4 cup crumbled feta cheese
1 tablespoon olive oil
Salt and pepper to taste

Instructions:

- Take a clean bowl, beat the eggs and season with salt and pepper.
- Over medium heat, cook olive oil in a non-stick skillet.
- Add spinach and tomatoes then cook for a minute.
- Pour the beaten eggs over the vegetables and cook until set.
- Sprinkle feta cheese on one half of the omelet, fold it over, and cook for another minute.
- Serve hot.

Total Calorie: 400

7. Mediterranean Shakshuka

Ingredients:

2 tablespoons olive oil
1 onion, thinly sliced
2 cloves garlic, minced
1 red bell pepper, sliced
1 can (400g) diced tomatoes
1 teaspoon ground cumin
1 teaspoon ground paprika
1/2 teaspoon ground cayenne pepper
4-6 large eggs
Salt and pepper to taste
Fresh parsley, chopped (for garnish)

Instructions:

- Preheat olive oil in a large pot or pan over medium heat.
- Pour in sliced onions and cook to softness, then add crushed garlic and fry for a minute.
- Add diced bell pepper and boil until tender.
- Pour in the diced tomatoes and spices (cumin, paprika, cayenne pepper) and seethe for 10-15 minutes.
- Dig sizable holes in the sauce and break the eggs into them.
- Cover the frypan and cook until the egg whites are set, but the yolks are still slushy (or cook longer if you prefer the yolks firm).

- Season with salt and pepper, garnish with chopped parsley, and serve with crusty bread.

Total Calories: 250

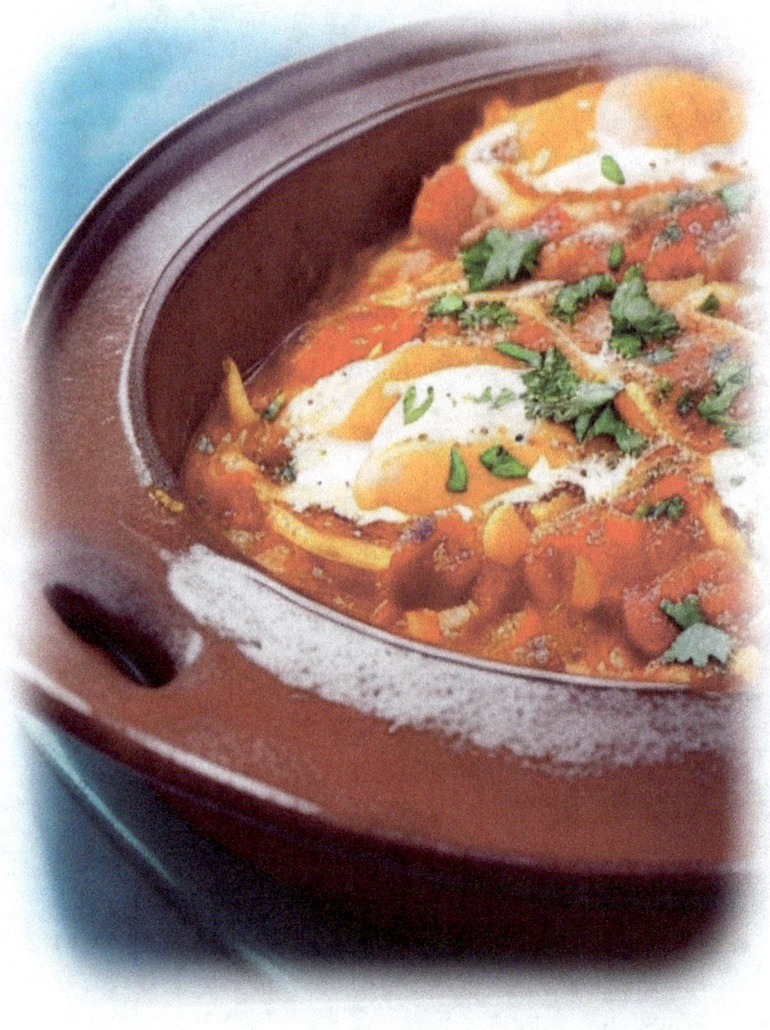

8. Mediterranean Fruit Salad

Ingredients:

1 cup diced watermelon
1 cup diced cantaloupe
1 cup diced honeydew melon
1 cup fresh strawberries, halved
1 tablespoon fresh mint leaves, chopped
1 tablespoon fresh lime juice
1 teaspoon honey (optional)

Instructions:

- In a large bowl, mix together all the diced fruits.
- In a small bowl, combine the lime juice and honey (if using) to create the dressing.
- Drizzle the dressing over the mixture and gently toss it to coat.
- Scatter the chopped mint leaves on top.
- Refrigerate for 10-15 minutes before serving.

Total Calories: 150

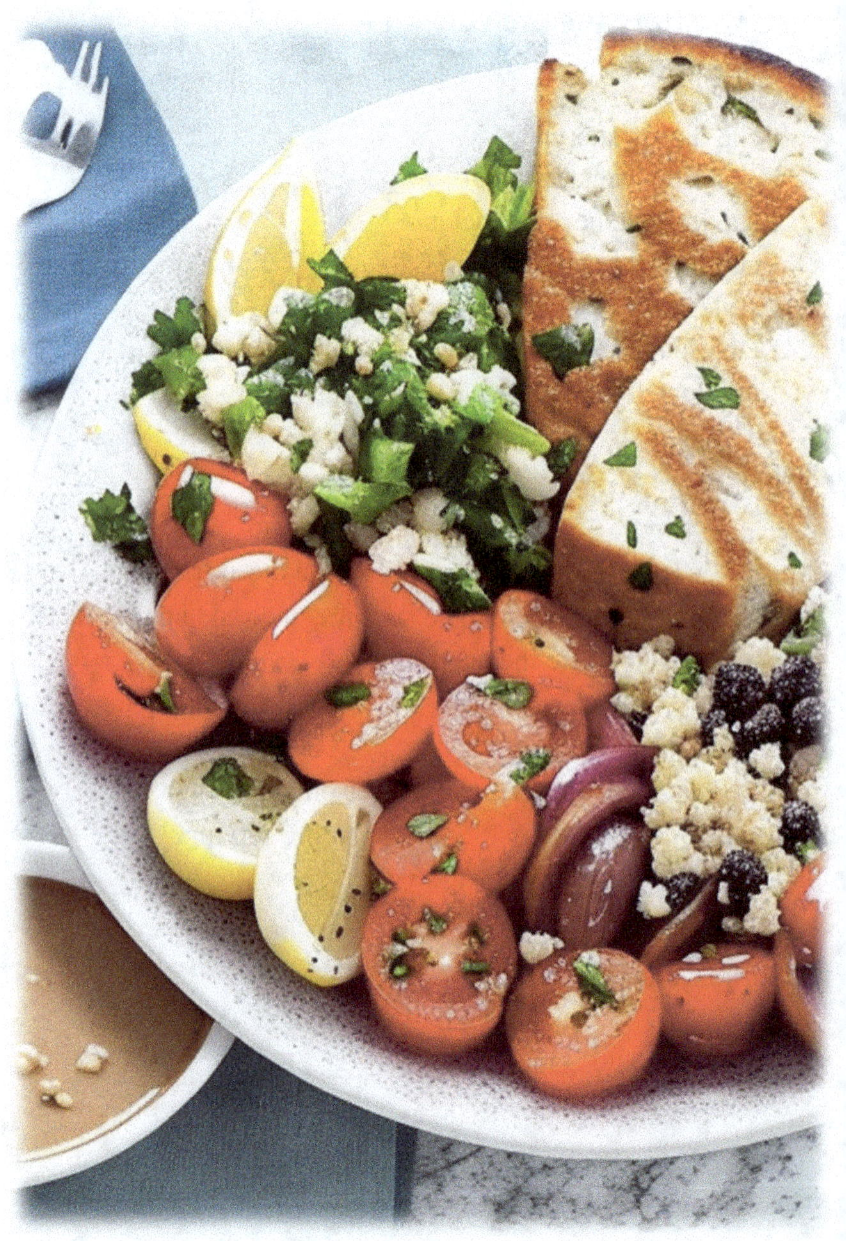

9. Mediterranean Breakfast Couscous

Ingredients:

1 cup cooked couscous
1/4 cup chopped dried apricots
1/4 cup chopped dates
2 tablespoons chopped pistachios
1 tablespoon honey
1/2 teaspoon ground cinnamon
1/4 cup Greek yogurt
Fresh mint leaves for garnish

Instructions:

- In a clean bowl, mix the cooked couscous with chopped dried apricots, dates, and pistachios.
- Drizzle honey over the couscous mixture and sprinkle ground cinnamon.
- Serve the couscous with a dollop of Greek yogurt on top.
- Garnish with fresh mint leaves.
- Mix the yogurt and couscous together before eating.

Total Calories: 350

10. Mediterranean Chia Seed Pudding

Ingredients:

1/4 cup chia seeds
1 cup almond milk (or any other milk of your choice)
1 tablespoon honey
1/2 teaspoon vanilla extract
1/4 cup fresh berries (blueberries, raspberries, strawberries)
1 tablespoon sliced almonds
Fresh mint leaves for garnish

Instructions:

- In a container or bowl, mix honey, chia seeds, almond milk, and vanilla extract.
- Stir well to perfectly mix all the ingredients.
- Cover the container and cool overnight or for at least 4 hours in a refrigerator. This enables the chia seeds to swell and form a pudding-like texture.
- Before serving, give the chia seed pudding a good stir.
- Top with fresh berries and sliced almonds.
- Garnish with fresh mint leaves.

Total Calories: 300

Lunch Recipes

1. Greek Salad

Ingredients:

2 cups romaine lettuce, chopped (20 cal)
1 cup cherry tomatoes, halved (60 cal)
1/2 cucumber, sliced (25 cal)
1/4 cup kalamata olives, pitted (70 cal)
1/4 red onion, thinly sliced (15 cal)
2 oz feta cheese, crumbled (110 cal)
2 Tbsp red wine vinegar (5 cal)
1 Tbsp olive oil (120 cal)
1 tsp oregano
Salt and pepper to taste

Instructions:

- Toss all ingredients together in a bowl.
- Add oregano, pepper, and salt to taste.

Total Calories: 425

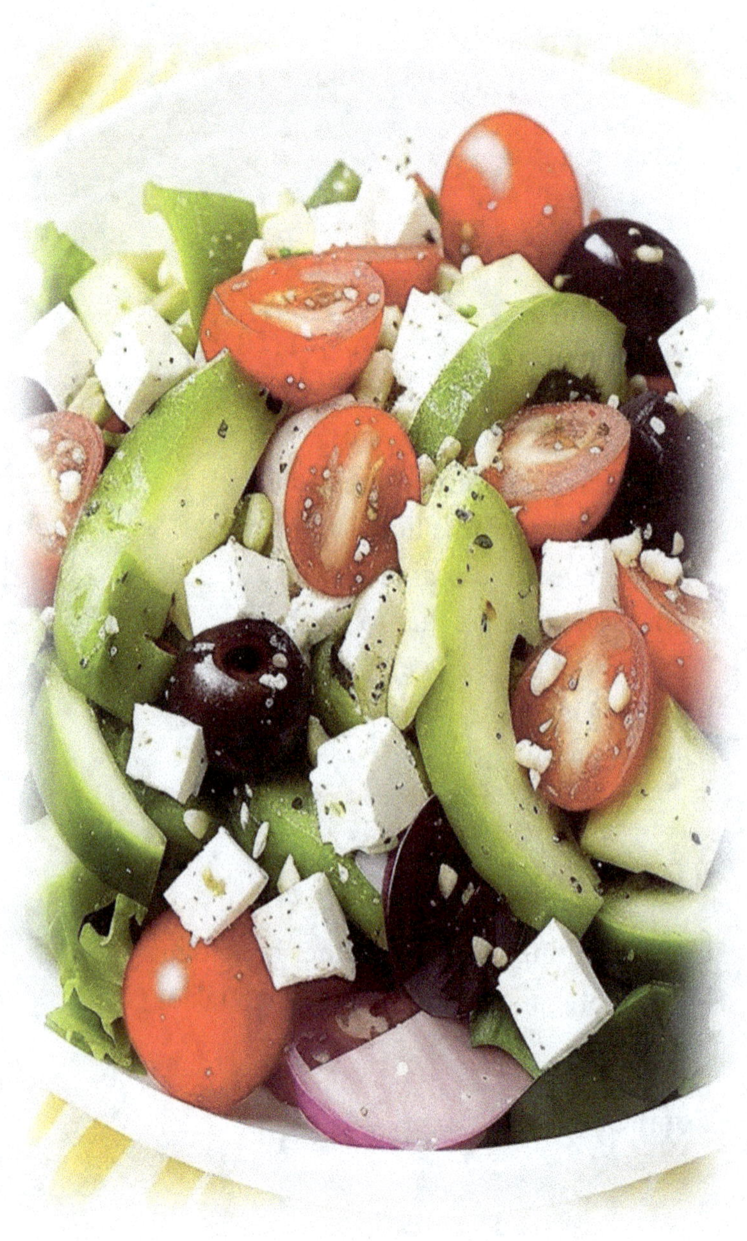

2. Tuna Salad Wraps

Ingredients:

5 oz canned tuna, drained (120 cal)
2 Tbsp plain Greek yogurt (17 cal)
1 celery stalk, diced (5 cal)
1 Tbsp lemon juice (5 cal)
1 tsp Dijon mustard
Salt and pepper to taste
2 whole wheat wraps (200 cal)

Instructions:

- Combine the tuna with yogurt, celery, lemon juice, and mustard.
- Add pepper and salt to taste.
- Spoon tuna salad onto each of the two whole wheat wraps.

Total Calories: 347

3. Mediterranean Quinoa Bowl

Ingredients:

1/2 cup quinoa, cooked (170 cal)
1/2 cup chickpeas, rinsed and drained (180 cal)
1/4 cup cherry tomatoes, halved (30 cal)
1/4 cucumber, diced (10 cal)
2 Tbsp crumbled feta cheese (55 cal)
2 Tbsp fresh parsley, chopped
2 Tbsp lemon juice (10 cal)
2 Tbsp olive oil (240 cal)
Salt and pepper to taste

Instructions:

- Quinoa, chickpeas, feta, parsley, tomatoes, cucumber, lemon juice, and olive oil should all be combined.
- Add pepper and salt to taste.

Total Calories: 695

4. Open-Faced Hummus Sandwiches

Ingredients:

4 slices whole grain bread (400 cal)
1/2 cup hummus (175 cal)
1 cup mixed greens (10 cal)
1/4 cucumber, sliced (10 cal)
2 Tbsp crumbled feta cheese (55 cal)
2 Tbsp olive oil (240 cal)
2 Tbsp balsamic vinegar (10 cal)

Instructions:

- Toast your bread.
- Cover each slice with hummus.
- Add feta, cucumber, and mixed greens on top.
- Finish with balsamic vinegar and olive oil drizzle.

Total Calories: 900

5. Lentil Vegetable Soup

Ingredients:

1 cup dried lentils, rinsed (230 cal)
6 cups vegetable broth (60 cal)
1 onion, diced (45 cal)
3 carrots, peeled and sliced (120 cal)
2 celery stalks, sliced (15 cal)
1 zucchini, diced (40 cal)
1 15-oz Can diced tomatoes (90 cal)
2 cloves garlic, minced
2 tsp oregano
Salt and pepper to taste

Instructions:

- All ingredients should be combined in a moderate pot.
- Allow it to cook for a while, then reduce the heat of the burner and simmer for 25 to 30 minutes, or until the lentils are tender.
- Add salt and pepper to taste.

Total Calories: 60

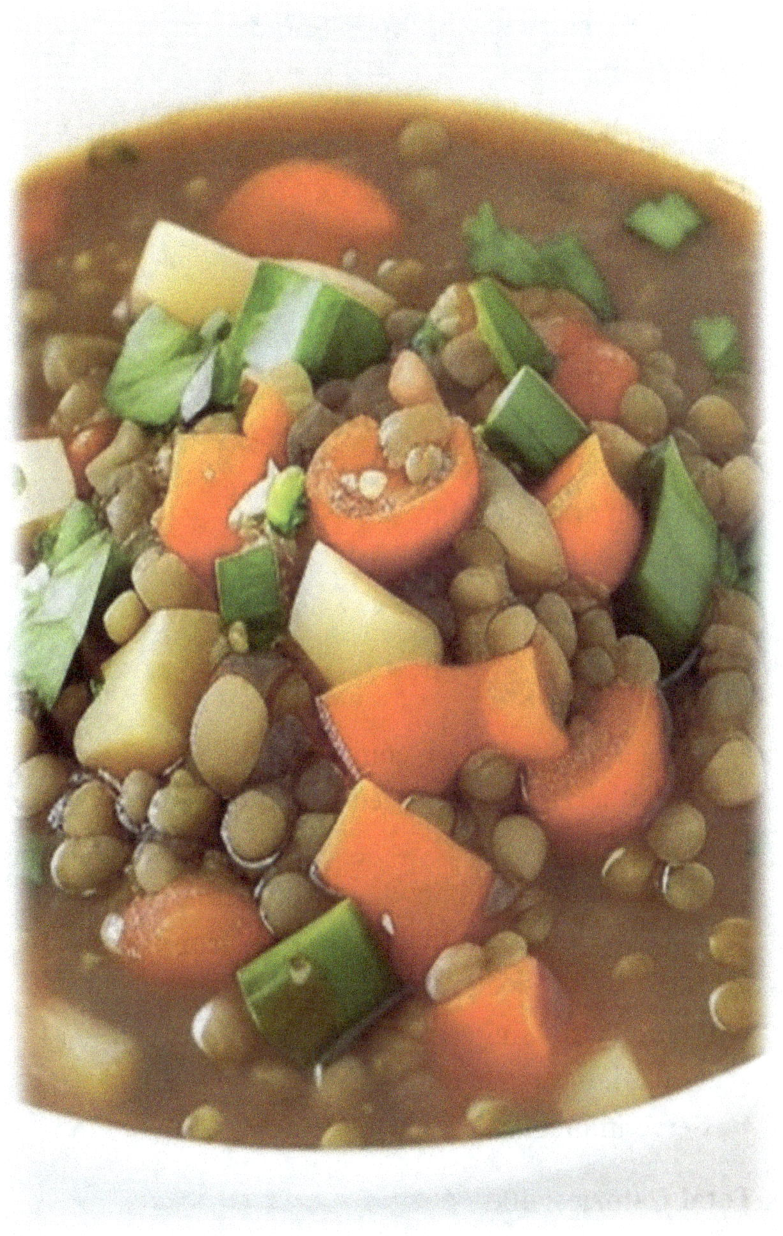

6. Mediterranean Chickpea Salad

Ingredients:

1 can (400g) chickpeas, drained and rinsed
1 cucumber, diced
1 bell pepper (any color), diced
1/4 cup chopped red onion
1/4 cup crumbled feta cheese
2 tablespoons chopped fresh parsley
2 tablespoons olive oil
1 tablespoon red wine vinegar
1 teaspoon dried oregano
Salt and pepper to taste

Instructions:

- In a large clean bowl, combine chickpeas, diced cucumber, bell pepper, red onion, feta cheese, and chopped parsley.
- In a separate small bowl, whisk together olive oil, red wine vinegar, dried oregano, salt, and pepper to make the dressing.
- Pour the dressing over the salad and toss gently to coat all ingredients.
- Serve immediately or refrigerate for later.

Total Calories: 400

7. Mediterranean Stuffed Peppers

Ingredients:

4 large bell peppers (any color)
1 cup cooked quinoa or couscous
1 can (400g) chickpeas, drained and rinsed
1 cup diced tomatoes
1/2 cup chopped Kalamata olives
1/4 cup crumbled feta cheese
2 tablespoons chopped fresh parsley
1 tablespoon olive oil
1 teaspoon ground cumin
Salt and pepper to taste

Instructions:

- Warm up the oven to 375°F (190°C).
- Slice off the top portion of the bell peppers and remove the membranes with the seeds.
- In a large bowl, mix cooked quinoa or couscous, chickpeas, diced tomatoes, Kalamata olives, feta cheese, chopped parsley, olive oil, ground cumin, salt, and pepper.
- Fill up the bell peppers using the quinoa mixture and arrange them properly in a baking dish.
- Cover the dish with foil and bake for about 25-30 minutes or until the peppers are tender.

- Serve steamy.

Total Calories: 400

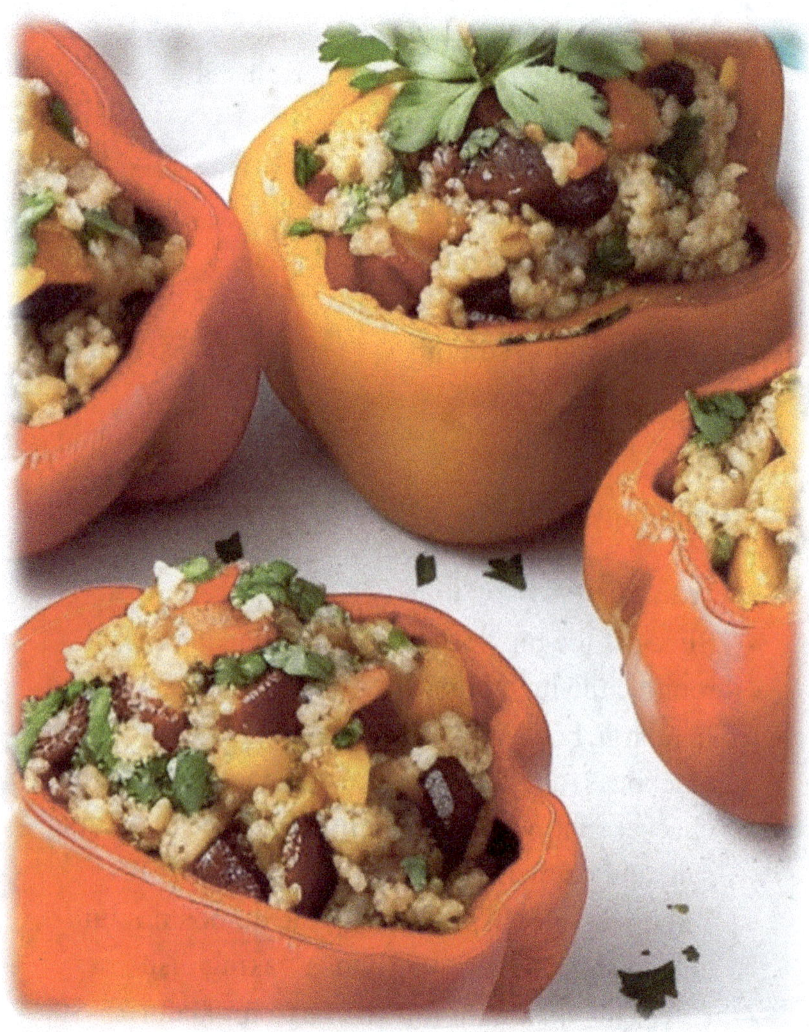

8. Mediterranean Spinach and Feta Stuffed Chicken

Ingredients:

4 boneless, skinless chicken breasts
1 cup chopped fresh spinach
1/2 cup crumbled feta cheese
1/4 cup chopped sun-dried tomatoes (packed in oil)
2 cloves garlic, minced
1 tablespoon olive oil
1 teaspoon dried oregano
Salt and pepper to taste
Lemon wedges for serving

Instructions:

- Heat up the oven to 375°F (190°C).
- In a bowl, mix chopped spinach, crumbled feta cheese, chopped sun-dried tomatoes, minced garlic, olive oil, dried oregano, salt, and pepper to make the stuffing.
- Carefully slice a pocket into each chicken breast.
- Insert the feta mixture and spinach into the parts of the chicken breasts.
- Place the stuffed chicken breasts in a baking dish.
- Bake for about 25-30 minutes or until the chicken is cooked through spand no longer pink in the center.

- You can serve it with lemon wedges placed tastefully on the side.

Total Calories: 400

9. Mediterranean Tuna Salad

Ingredients:

2 cans (5 oz each) tuna, drained
1/2 cup diced cucumber
1/2 cup diced cherry tomatoes
1/4 cup chopped red onion
1/4 cup pitted Kalamata olives, chopped
2 tablespoons chopped fresh parsley
2 tablespoons lemon juice
1 tablespoon olive oil
1 teaspoon dried oregano
Salt and pepper to taste
Whole grain pita bread or lettuce leaves for serving

Instructions:

- In a large clean bowl, mix tuna, diced cucumber, cherry tomatoes, red onion, chopped Kalamata olives, and fresh parsley.
- Using another smaller bowl, turn together lemon juice, pepper, olive oil, dried oregano, and salt to form the dressing.
- Empty the dressing over the tuna mixture and turn gently to blend.

- Serve the Mediterranean tuna salad in whole grain pita bread or wrapped in lettuce leaves.

Total Calories: 350

10. Mediterranean Shrimp and Orzo Salad

Ingredients:

8 oz (225g) cooked shrimp, peeled and deveined
1 cup cooked orzo pasta
1/2 cup cherry tomatoes, halved
1/4 cup crumbled feta cheese
1/4 cup pitted Kalamata olives, halved
2 tablespoons chopped fresh basil
2 tablespoons lemon juice
1 tablespoon olive oil
Salt and pepper to taste

Instructions:

- In a large bowl, combine cooked shrimp, cooked orzo pasta, halved cherry tomatoes, crumbled feta cheese, halved Kalamata olives, and chopped fresh basil.
- With a smaller bowl, mix olive oil, lemon juice, pepper, and salt to create the dressing.
- Pour the dressing over the salad and toss gently to combine all ingredients.
- Serve at room temperature or chilled.

Total Calories: 400

Dinner Recipes

1. Ratatouille

Ingredients:

1 onion, sliced (45 cal)
1 eggplant, diced (35 cal)
1 zucchini, sliced (40 cal)
1 red pepper, sliced (50 cal)
3 cloves garlic, minced (15 cal)
14 oz can dice tomatoes (90 cal)
2 Tbsp olive oil (240 cal)
1 tsp dried thyme
Basil leaves for garnish

Instructions:

- The onion should be fried in oil.
- Cook for five minutes after adding pepper, thyme, zucchini, and eggplant.
- Garlic and tomatoes should be added, and the sauce should be allowed to simmer for 20 minutes to thicken.
- Basil is a good garnish.

Total Calories: 515

2. Shrimp Scampi

Ingredients:

12 jumbo shrimp, peeled (120 cal)
3 cloves garlic, minced (15 cal)
1 lemon, juiced (15 cal)
1/4 cup dry white wine (70 cal)
2 Tbsp olive oil (240 cal)
1 lb whole wheat linguine (440 cal)
2 Tbsp parsley, chopped

Instructions:

- Follow the instructions on the pasta's package to cook it.
- Garlic and shrimp should be sauteed in oil.
- The fried shrimp should be simmered with wine and lemon juice until they turn pink.
- Combine pasta and parsley.

Total Calories: 900

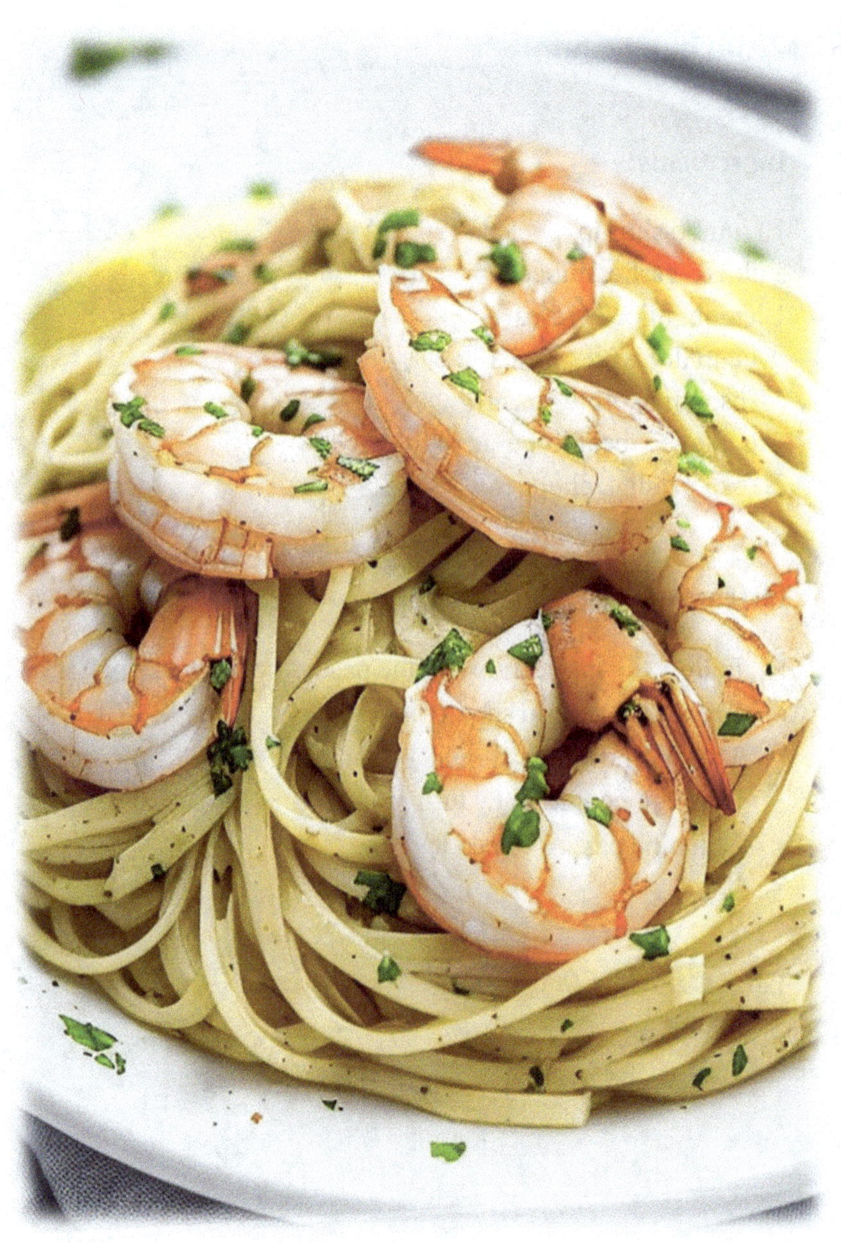

3. Greek Stuffed Peppers

Ingredients:

4 bell peppers, halved and seeded (80 cal)
1 cup cooked quinoa (170 cal)
1 cup cooked chickpeas (270 cal)
1/4 cup crumbled feta cheese (110 cal)
1/4 cup kalamata olives, chopped (70 cal)
2 Tbsp fresh dill, chopped
2 Tbsp lemon juice (10 cal)
2 Tbsp olive oil (240 cal)

Instructions:

- Heat the oven to about a temperature of 400 degrees Fahrenheit.
- Combine quinoa, chickpeas, feta, olives, dill, and lemon juice with oil.
- The mixture should be divided among pepper halves.
- Bake peppers for 30 minutes, or until they are soft.

Total Calories: 950

4. Seafood Paella

Ingredients:

2 Tbsp olive oil (240 cal)
1 onion, diced (45 cal)
3 garlic cloves, minced (15 cal)
1 cup short grain rice, cooked (440 cal)
1/2 tsp saffron threads
1 cup tomato sauce (70 cal)
3 cups seafood stock (105 cal)
12 mussels, scrubbed (150 cal)
12 clams, scrubbed (120 cal)
12 shrimp, peeled (120 cal)
1/4 cup parsley, chopped

Instructions:

- Sauté onion and garlic in hot oil.
- Add the rice, then stir for one minute.
- Stock, tomato sauce, shrimp, clams, and saffron should be added.
- Add seafood to rice during the final five minutes of simmering to make it tender.
- Add some parsley as a garnish.

Total Calories: 1,325

5. Eggplant Parmesan

Ingredients:

1 large eggplant, sliced into rounds (75 cal)
1 cup breadcrumbs (140 cal)
1/2 cup Parmesan, grated (220 cal)
2 eggs, beaten (140 cal)
2 cups marinara sauce (150 cal)
1/4 cup fresh basil, chopped
1 lb whole wheat spaghetti (440 cal)

Instructions:

- Breadcrumbs and eggplant slices should be mixed with egg.
- Fry until golden in olive oil.
- In a baking dish, arrange the cheese, sauce, and fried eggplant.
- Bake it for 30 minutes.
- Toss basil on top before serving over pasta.

Total Calories: 1,165

6. Seafood Paella

Ingredients:

2 Tbsp olive oil (240 cal)
6 boneless skinless chicken thighs, diced (1080 cal)
1 onion, diced (45 cal)
4 cloves garlic, minced (20 cal)
1 red bell pepper, sliced (50 cal)
1 cup short grain rice (440 cal)
1 tsp smoked paprika
1 14oz can diced tomatoes (90 cal)
3 cups chicken broth (105 cal)
12 jumbo shrimp, peeled (120 cal)
1/4 cup parsley, chopped

Instructions:

- Warm oil in a pan.
- Fry the chicken and onion until the chicken browns.
- Include the broth, rice, paprika, tomatoes, garlic, and pepper.
- Add shrimp to the pot five minutes before the rice is ready to be served.
- Use parsley for garnish.

Total Calories: 2,190

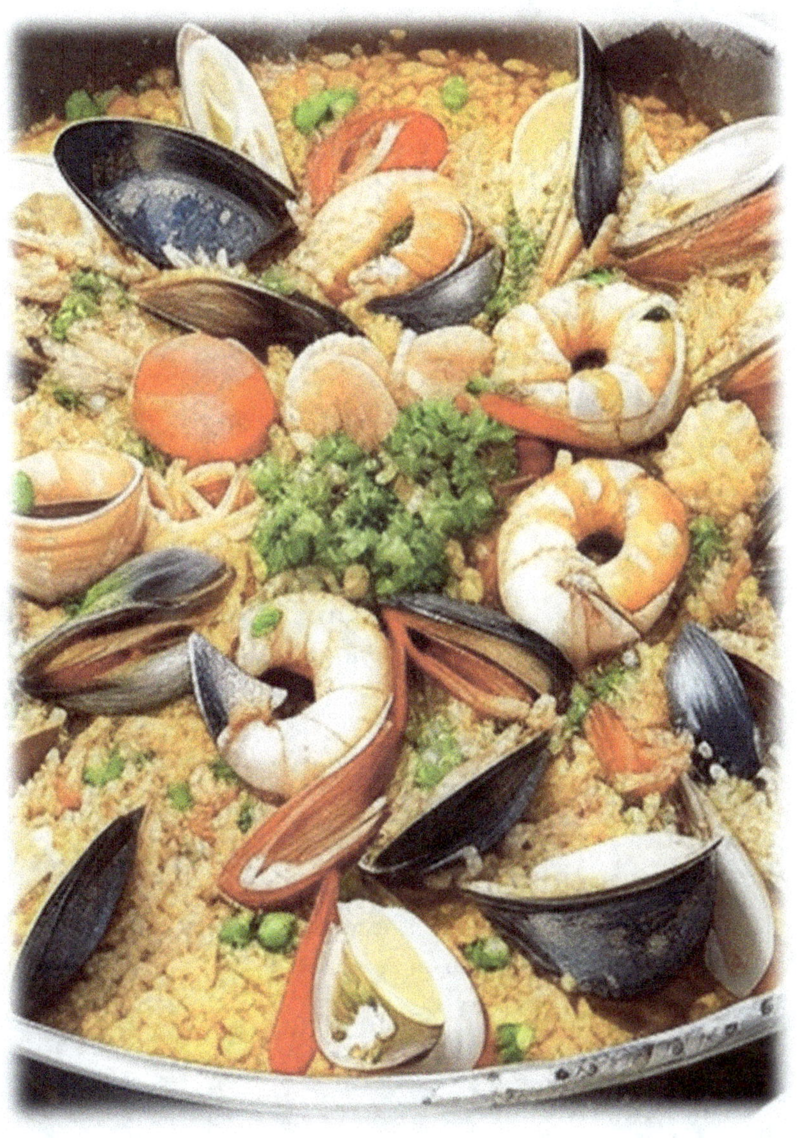

7. Mediterranean Grilled Fish

Ingredients:

4 fish fillets (such as salmon, sea bass, or cod)
2 tablespoons olive oil
2 cloves garlic, minced
1 tablespoon lemon juice
1 teaspoon dried oregano
1 teaspoon dried thyme
Salt and pepper to taste
Lemon wedges for serving

Instructions:

- In a small bowl, mix olive oil, minced garlic, lemon juice, dried oregano, dried thyme, salt, and pepper to make the marinade.
- Coat the fish fillets with the marinade and let them sit for at least 20 minutes.
- Preheat the grill to medium-high heat.
- Place the fish on the grill to roast for about 3-4 minutes on both sides or until it becomes properly cooked.
- Serve with lemon wedges.

Total Calories: 300

8. Mediterranean Lemon Herb Chicken

Ingredients:

4 boneless, skinless chicken breasts
2 tablespoons olive oil
Zest and juice of 1 lemon
2 cloves garlic, minced
1 teaspoon dried oregano
1 teaspoon dried thyme
Salt and pepper to taste
Fresh parsley for garnish

Instructions:

- In a bowl, mix olive oil, lemon zest, lemon juice, minced garlic, dried oregano, dried thyme, salt, and pepper to create the marinade.
- Add chicken breasts to the marinade and coat them evenly.
- Cover the bowl and let the chicken marinate in the refrigerator for at least 30 minutes.
- Preheat the oven to 375°F (190°C).
- Place the marinated chicken in a baking dish and bake for about 25-30 minutes or until the chicken is cooked through.
- Garnish with fresh parsley before serving.

Total Calories: 300

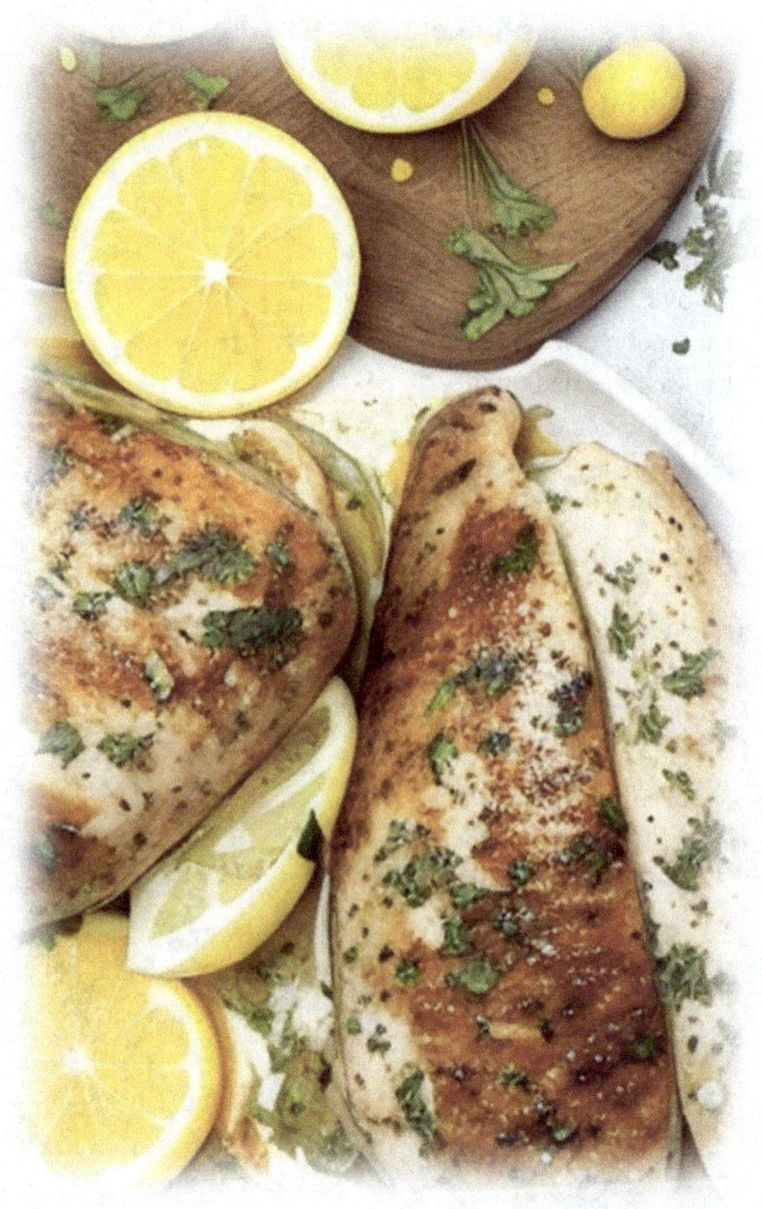

9. Mediterranean Shrimp and Tomato Pasta

Ingredients:

8 oz (225g) whole wheat spaghetti or linguine
1 lb (450g) skinned and deveined large shrimp
2 tablespoons olive oil
3 cloves garlic, minced
1 can (400g) diced tomatoes
1/4 cup pitted Kalamata olives, chopped
1/4 cup chopped fresh basil
1/2 teaspoon dried red pepper flakes (optional)
Salt and pepper to taste
Grated Parmesan cheese for serving

Instructions:

- Boil the pasta by following the instructions on the package. Drain out the water and set it aside.
- In a clean cooking pot, warm up the olive oil using medium heat.
- At this point, add the minced garlic and fry it for one minute or until fragrant.
- Now, throw in the shrimp and stir-fry until it becomes opaque.
- Stir in the diced tomatoes, chopped Kalamata olives, fresh basil, dried red pepper flakes (if using), salt, and pepper.
- Allow it to simmer for 5 to 6 minutes or until the sauce becomes slightly thickened.

- Add the cooked pasta to the skillet and toss it with the shrimp and tomato sauce until well combined.
- You can add grated Parmesan cheese on top while serving.

Total Calories: 450

10. Mediterranean Grilled Vegetable Platter

Ingredients:

1 eggplant, sliced
1 zucchini, sliced lengthwise
1 yellow squash, sliced lengthwise
1 red bell pepper, halved and deseeded
1 red onion, sliced into thick rounds
1 tablespoon olive oil
2 cloves garlic, minced
1 tablespoon balsamic vinegar
1 teaspoon dried oregano
Salt and pepper to taste
Fresh basil leaves for garnish

Instructions:

- Preheat the grill to medium-high heat.
- In a large bowl, toss the sliced vegetables with olive oil, minced garlic, balsamic vinegar, dried oregano, salt, and pepper.
- Grill the vegetables for about 3-4 minutes per side or until they have nice grill marks and are tender.
- Arrange the grilled vegetables on a platter and garnish with fresh basil leaves before serving.

Total Calories: 250

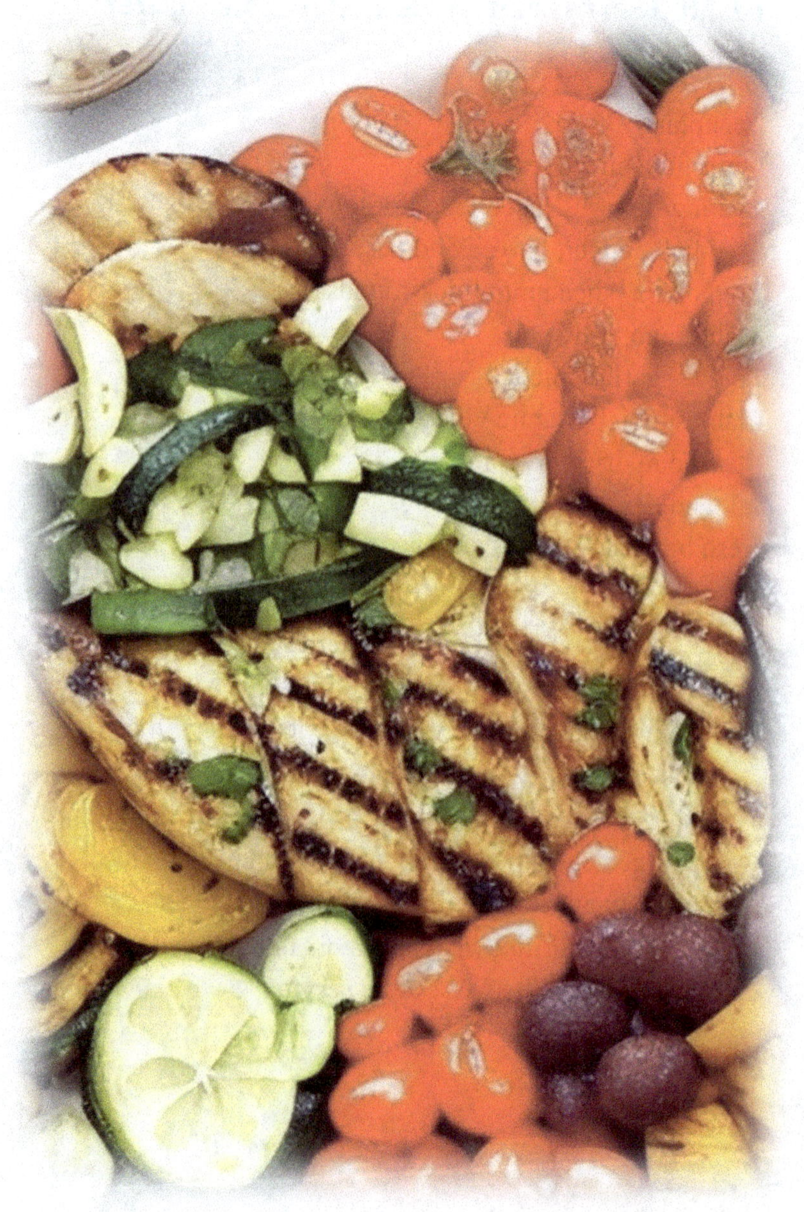

11. Mediterranean Stuffed Eggplant

Ingredients:

2 large eggplants
1 cup cooked couscous
1/2 cup diced tomatoes
1/4 cup chopped Kalamata olives
1/4 cup crumbled feta cheese
2 tablespoons chopped fresh parsley
2 tablespoons olive oil
1 tablespoon lemon juice
1 teaspoon ground cumin
Salt and pepper to taste

Instructions:

- Preheat the oven to 375°F (190°C).
- Cut the eggplants in half lengthwise and scoop out the flesh to create a hollow center.
- In a large bowl, mix cooked couscous, diced tomatoes, chopped Kalamata olives, crumbled feta cheese, chopped parsley, olive oil, lemon juice, ground cumin, salt, and pepper.
- Stuff the eggplant halves with the couscous mixture.
- Place the eggplant halves you stuffed in a baking dish.
- Cover the dish with foil and bake for about 25-30 minutes or until the eggplant is tender and the filling is heated through.

Total Calories: 400

Appetizers and Snacks

1. Tzatziki Dip

Ingredients:

1 cucumber, grated and drained (25 cal)
1 cup Greek yogurt (150 cal)
3 cloves garlic, minced (15 cal)
2 Tbsp olive oil (240 cal)
2 Tbsp lemon juice (10 cal)
1 tsp dill
Salt and pepper to taste

Instructions:

- Combine cucumber, yogurt, dill, garlic, olive oil, and lemon juice.
- Add pepper and salt to taste.
- Serve together with fresh vegetables or pita chips.

Total Calories: 440

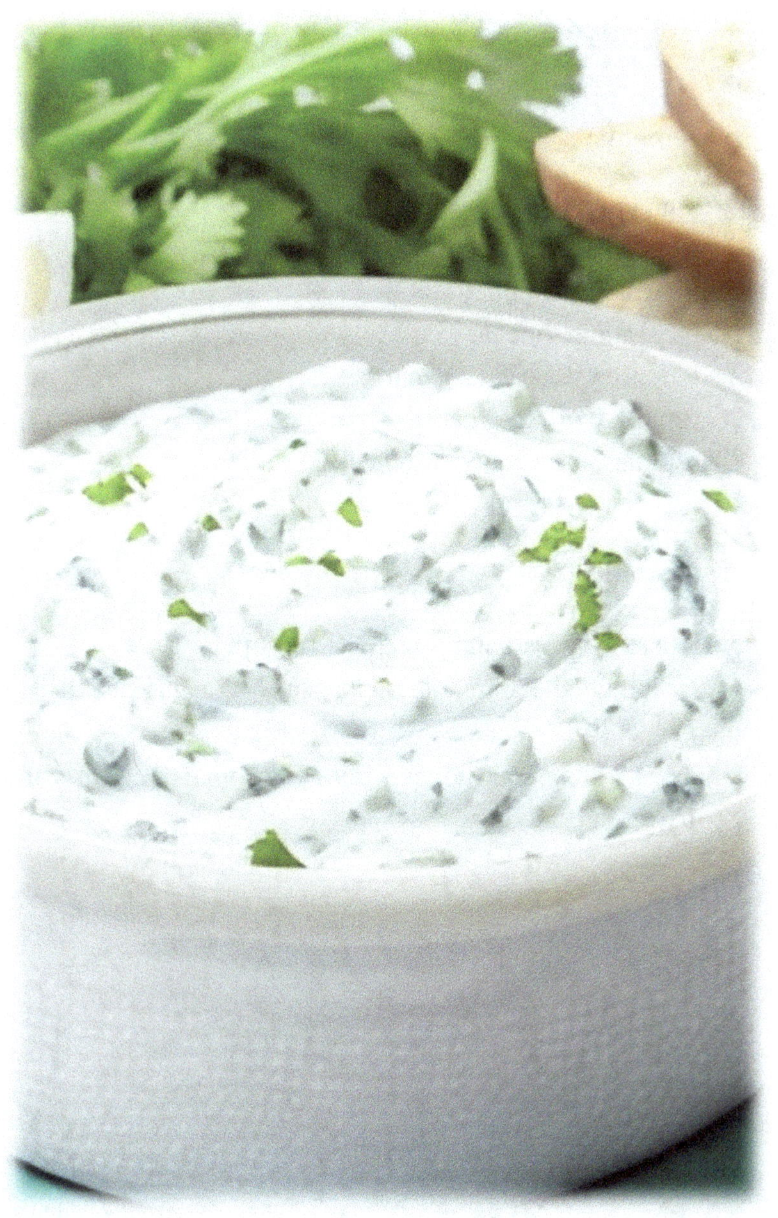

2. Tomato & Basil Bruschetta

Ingredients:

2 Roma tomatoes, diced (30 cal)
1 garlic clove, minced (5 cal)
5 basil leaves, chopped
1 tsp balsamic vinegar (5 cal)
2 slices crusty bread (200 cal)
2 Tbsp olive oil (240 cal)
2 Tbsp parmesan, shaved (60 cal)

Instructions:

- Toast the bread and drizzle it with oil.
- Combine the tomatoes, , balsamic vinegar, basil, and garlic.
- Toasts should be topped with the tomato mixture and parmesan shavings.

Total Calories: 540

3. Marinated Olives

Ingredients:

1 cup mixed olives, drained (140 cal)
1 garlic clove, sliced
1 tsp fresh thyme
1 tsp lemon zest
2 Tbsp olive oil (240 cal)
1 Tbsp red wine vinegar (5 cal)

Instructions:

- Combine olives, garlic, thyme, lemon zest, olive oil, and vinegar.
- With at least 30 minutes for it to marinate before serving.

Total Calories: 385

4. Baba Ganoush

Ingredients:

1 large eggplant, roasted (75 cal)
2 Tbsp tahini (90 cal)
1 lemon, juiced (15 cal)
1 garlic clove, minced (5 cal)
2 Tbsp olive oil (240 cal)
2 Tbsp parsley, chopped
Salt and pepper to taste

Instructions:

- Scrape the flesh of the roasted eggplant into a bowl.
- Combine with parsley, tahini, garlic, lemon juice, and olive oil.
- Add salt and pepper to taste.
- Accompany it with veggies or pita.

Total Calories: 425

5. Caprese Skewers

Ingredients:

12 cherry tomatoes (60 cal)
12 basil leaves
12 bocconcini balls, drained (300 cal)
2 Tbsp balsamic glaze (40 cal)

Instructions:

- Skewer tomatoes, basil leaves, and bocconcini balls.
- Add a glaze of balsamic vinegar and serve.

Total Calories: 400

Desserts

1. Yogurt with Honey & Walnuts

Ingredients:

- 1 cup Greek yogurt (150 cal)
- 1 Tbsp honey (60 cal)
- 1/4 cup walnuts, chopped (200 cal)

Instructions:

Top yogurt with drizzled honey and chopped walnuts.

Total Calories: 410

2. Crème Brûlée

Ingredients:

2 cups heavy cream (1600 cal)
1 vanilla bean, split and scraped
6 egg yolks (420 cal)
1/2 cup sugar, divided (200 cal)

Instructions:

- Cream and vanilla should be simmered.
- Mix 1/4 cup sugar and yolks until they are light in color.
- As you whisk, add hot cream.
- Pour into some ramekins and bake at 325°F for 25–30 minutes.
- Allow to cool a bit, then add a layer of sugar and caramelize.

Total Calories: 2220

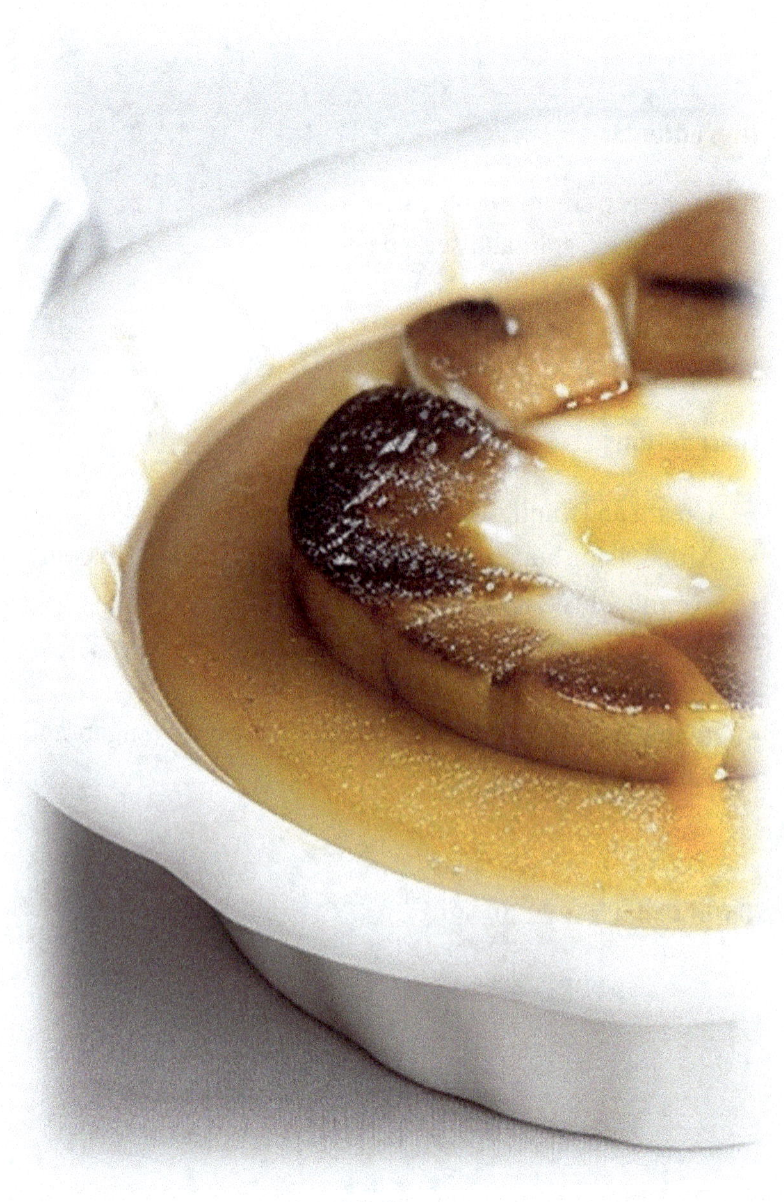

3. Lemon Ricotta Cake

Ingredients:

2 cups ricotta cheese (720 cal)
1/2 cup sugar (200 cal)
2 eggs (140 cal)
Zest of 2 lemons
2/3 cup flour (240 cal)
1 tsp baking powder

Lemon glaze:
1/3 cup lemon juice (15 cal)
1/2 cup powdered sugar (200 cal)

Instructions:

- Mix ricotta, sugar, eggs, and lemon zest.
- Flour and baking powder should be added and properly combined.
- Move the mix to a greased pan and bake at 375°F for 45 to 50 minutes.
- Combine powdered sugar and lemon juice to make a glaze.

Total Calories: 1515

4. Walnut & Orange Cake

Ingredients:

1 1/2 cups walnuts, chopped (1050 cal)
1 cup sugar (400 cal)
2 eggs (140 cal)
Zest of 1 orange
2/3 cup flour (240 cal)
1 tsp baking powder
1/4 tsp salt

Instructions:

- Finely process walnuts using a food processor.
- Add sugar, eggs, and orange zest by whisking.
- Mix with salt, baking soda, and flour.
- Bake for 30-35 minutes at 350F.

Total Calories: 1830

5. Fig & Walnut Loaf

Ingredients:

1 cup figs, diced (260 cal)
1/2 cup walnuts, chopped (400 cal)
Zest of 1 orange
1 3/4 cups flour (620 cal)
3/4 cup sugar (300 cal)
1 tsp baking soda
1/2 cup plain Greek yogurt (75 cal)
2 eggs (140 cal)
1/3 cup olive oil (400 cal)

Instructions:

- Mix the figs, walnuts, zest, flour, sugar, and baking soda.
- Add the yogurt, eggs, and oil, and mix everything until they are properly combined.
- Bake at 350F for 50 to 60 minutes.

Total Calories: 2195

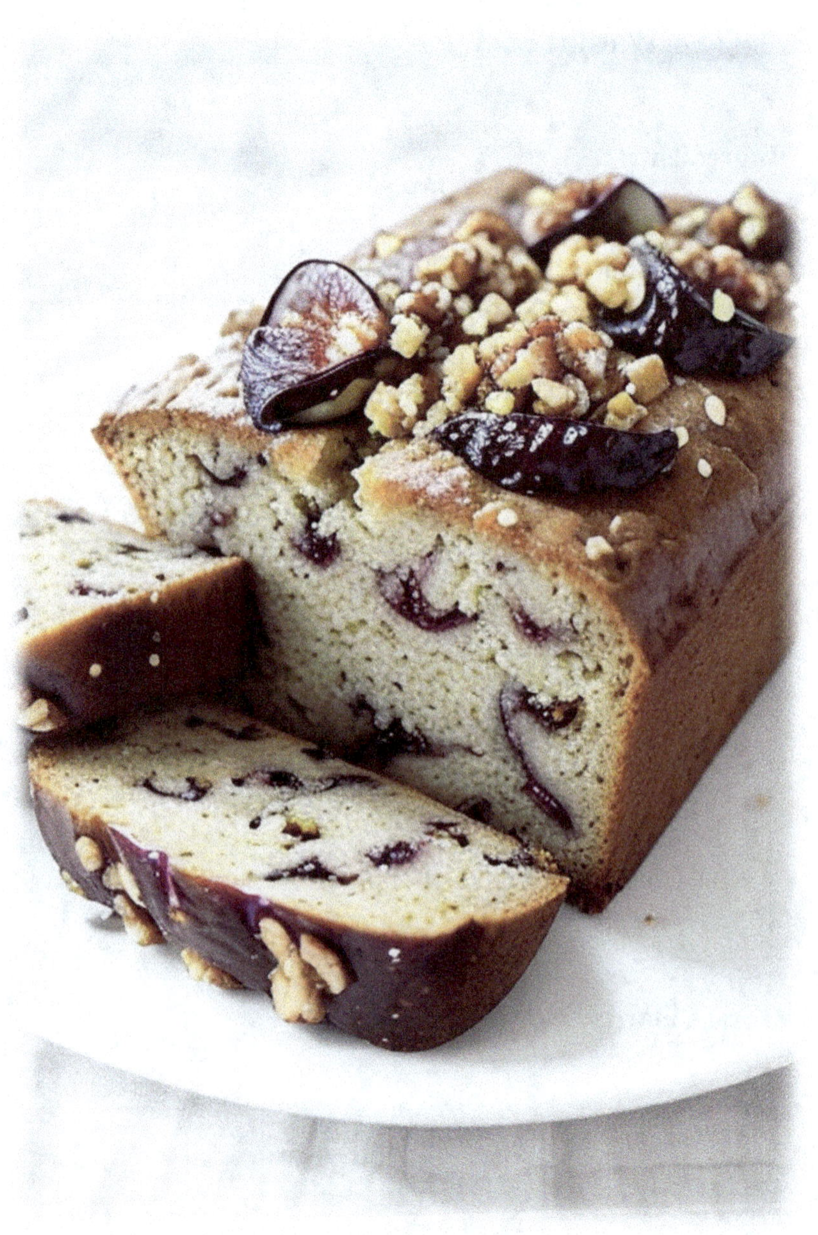

CONCLUSION

And that sums up our delightful voyage through the colorful tastes of the Mediterranean! I sincerely hope you enjoy these recipes as much as I enjoyed creating them and sharing the wonder of this nutritious, delectable meal with you.

Cooking these recipes has shown me personally the delight that cuisine created from basic, nutritious ingredients can bring to the table.

Meals become less about luxury and more about camaraderie when plant-based cuisine takes center stage. A plate of roasted vegetables, a bowl of lentils, or a crusty loaf of bread brushed with olive oil can all bring you a lot of happiness.

My sincere appreciation for allowing me to be your guide to the Mediterranean kitchen. It has been an honor to share bread with you all if only symbolically speaking.

I wish you many wonderful experiences preparing dishes from this book and welcome you to make them your own. I'd love to read your ratings and reviews of the book on Amazon.

Most of all, I hope every dish encourages you to slow down and relish both your food and your loved ones gathered around the table. That is the genuine essence of the Mediterranean lifestyle. And thus, from my kitchen to yours, till we cook again - bye for now.

28 Days Meal Plan

Week 1	Breakfast	Lunch	Dinner
Monday	Avocado Toast	Greek Salad	Shrimp Scampi
Tuesday	Overnight Oats	Mediterranean Quinoa Bowl	Eggplant Parmesan
Wednesday	Mediterranean Omelets	Lentil Vegetable Soup	Mediterranean Lemon Herb Chicken
Thursday	Mediterranean Shakshuka	Open-Faced Hummus Sandwiches	Seafood Paella
Friday	Breakfast Tacos	Mediterranean Chickpea Salad	Ratatouille
Saturday	Vegetable Frittata	Mediterranean Stuffed Peppers	Mediterranean Grilled Fish
Sunday	Greek Yogurt Bowl	Tuna Salad Wraps	Mediterranean Shrimp and Tomato Pasta

Week 2	Breakfast	Lunch	Dinner
Monday	Mediterranean Fruit Salad	Mediterranean Spinach and Feta Stuffed Chicken	Mediterranean Stuffed Eggplant
Tuesday	Mediterranean Breakfast Couscous	Mediterranean Tuna Salad	Mediterranean Lemon Garlic Shrimp Pasta
Wednesday	Mediterranean Chia Seed Pudding	Greek Salad	Eggplant Parmesan
Thursday	Avocado Toast	Mediterranean Quinoa Bowl	Mediterranean Grilled Vegetable Platter
Friday	Overnight Oats	Lentil Vegetable Soup	Seafood Paella
Saturday	Mediterranean Omelets	Open-Faced Hummus Sandwiches	Shrimp Scampi
Sunday	Mediterranean Shakshuka	Mediterranean Chickpea Salad	Ratatouille

Week 3	Breakfast	Lunch	Dinner
Monday	Breakfast Tacos	Tuna Salad Wraps	Mediterranean Lemon Herb Chicken
Tuesday	Vegetable Frittata	Mediterranean Stuffed Peppers	Mediterranean Grilled Fish
Wednesday	Greek Yogurt Bowl	Greek Salad	Mediterranean Shrimp and Tomato Pasta
Thursday	Mediterranean Fruit Salad	Mediterranean Spinach and Feta Stuffed Chicken	Mediterranean Stuffed Eggplant
Friday	Mediterranean Breakfast Couscous	Mediterranean Tuna Salad	Mediterranean Lemon Garlic Shrimp Pasta
Saturday	Mediterranean Chia Seed Pudding	Greek Salad	Eggplant Parmesan
Sunday	Avocado Toast	Mediterranean Quinoa Bowl	Mediterranean Grilled Vegetable Platter

Week 4	Breakfast	Lunch	Dinner
Monday	Overnight Oats	Lentil Vegetable Soup	Seafood Paella
Tuesday	Mediterranean Omelets	Open-Faced Hummus Sandwiches	Shrimp Scampi
Wednesday	Mediterranean Shakshuka	Mediterranean Chickpea Salad	Ratatouille
Thursday	Breakfast Tacos	Tuna Salad Wraps	Mediterranean Lemon Herb Chicken
Friday	Vegetable Frittata	Mediterranean Stuffed Peppers	Mediterranean Grilled Fish
Saturday	Greek Yogurt Bowl	Greek Salad	Mediterranean Shrimp and Tomato Pasta
Sunday	Mediterranean Fruit Salad	Mediterranean Spinach and Feta Stuffed Chicken	Mediterranean Stuffed Eggplant

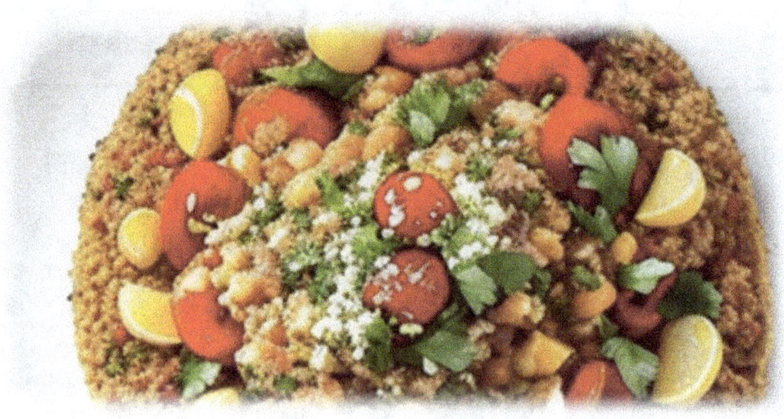

Thank you for letting me be your guide into this nourishing way of eating and living.

I wish you many happy, healthy years around the table! May your days be filled with good food, laughter and togetherness. Now go spread the Mediterranean spirit!